The Caring Person's Guide to Handling the Severely Multiply Handicapped

Rachel Golding
and
Liz Goldsmith

Illustrations by Martin Battye

MACMILLAN

First published 1986

Published by
MACMILLAN EDUCATION LTD
Houndmills, Basingstoke, Hampshire RG21 2XS
and London
Companies and representatives
throughout the world

Printed by Tisbury Printing, Salisbury

British Library Cataloguing in Publication Data
Golding, R.
The caring person's guide to handling the
severely multiply handicapped.
1. Handicapped——Care and treatment
I. Title   II. Goldsmith, L.
362.4   HV1568
ISBN 0–333–38619–1

Contents

Foreword

This guide is by practitioners in the Mental Handicap Service for practitioners in that service. It is a guide that demands a response from those who read it and in this way the lives of many mentally handicapped people will improve and the deformities seen so often in our long-stay wards will be minimised and possibly prevented in future generations.

In the past, it has proved difficult to attract Psychologists and Physiotherapists into the Mental Handicap Service. What could be done for mentally handicapped adults? Surely profoundly handicapped people do not present a therapeutic challenge? An attitude of therapeutic nihilism and custodial inactivity was prevalent and many profoundly handicapped people with unnecessary handicaps spent their lives without purpose or happiness.

This activity guide, written by a Clinical Psychologist and a Physiotherapist, both of whom have extensive experience with profoundly and multiply handicapped people, is for anyone who looks after such a person, and is to help them to use their time and skills more effectively, to minimise or prevent deformities and to position the person advantageously for his well-being and development. The guide is in several sections, the design being based on problem orientation so that the user can work through, answer the questions, seek for the next piece of information and finally decide on the optimal means of intervention.

Much of the time of a Physiotherapist in the Mental Handicap Service is rightly spent in increasing the skills in physical care of other caring staff and the parents. This guide will greatly support that endeavour, allowing those who are untrained in physical care to be sure of the aims of treatment, to avoid harmful interventions and choose those that will maximise the limited skills of the mentally handicapped person.

Attitudes to profoundly handicapped people are still tinged with pessimism. This guide will help to make progress with the treatment of profoundly handicapped people; it will help to convince both ourselves as well as others that improvements are possible and that good physical care is the basis for all other areas of development. The authors are to be congratulated on the production of a guide which will have far-reaching effects in improving the lives of those who present us with so many challenges.

Joan Bicknell
Professor of the Psychiatry
of Mental Handicap

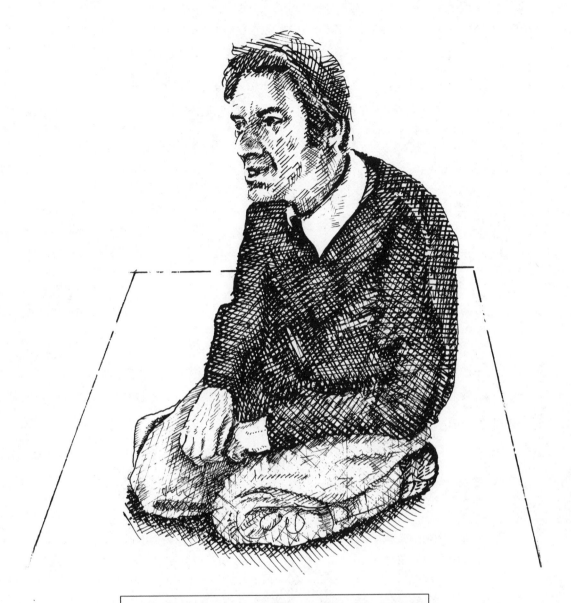

'How best to care for the multiply handicapped, and how to enable them to live lives that
are as rich and meaningful as possible, has
...... become not merely an ethical, psycho-
logical and nursing problem affecting only a
few, but also a social problem affecting sub-
stantial numbers of people.'

(Prof. J. Tizard in his Foreword to
Maureen Oswin (1978). *Children Living in Long Stay
Hospitals*,
Spastics International Medical Publications,
Research Monograph 5,
Heinemann, London)

Information

Name of patient _____

Date of birth _____

Address _____

_____

_____

Attendance at school, ATC, etc. (please specify place attended and time) _____

_____

If your patient lives in hospital, date of admission _____

_____

Name of key worker _____

Name of co-worker _____

Physiotherapist _____

Other professionals involved (e.g. doctor, teacher, psychologist, social worker, occupational

therapist, etc.) _____

_____

_____

_____

_____

_____

_____

_____

_____

Introduction to the Guide

Why has this Guide been Written?

This guide has been written to help anyone working with the severely multiply handicapped to be able to do the following:

1. **Learn how to identify the physical problems of the patient.**

   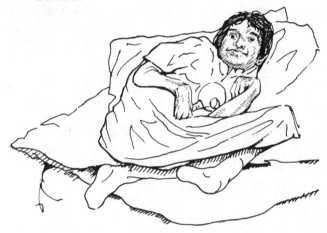

2. **Discover how these problems affect the patient and what will happen if they are not treated.**

3. **Find out what methods could be used to treat some of these problems.**

   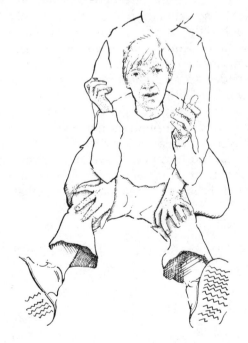

4. **Develop a plan of action whereby the needs which have been identified are met.**

   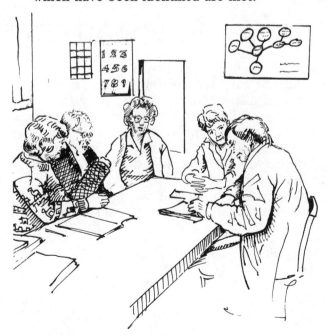

This guide is not designed to reduce the need for a physiotherapist but rather to enable the care giver and physiotherapist to communicate more effectively for the patient's benefit.

Your patient is likely to have many problems that are associated with his physical and mental handicaps and are not covered in this guide. For example, he may need special help with feeding, he may have behaviour problems, he may have difficulty in hearing or seeing.

Your patient's emotional, social and educational needs are of no less importance than his physical care.

However, good physical management provides a sound foundation for work on these additional areas of need and should increase the chances of success. For example, a good sitting position and correct support make feeding easier; certain positions and aids make it possible for the patient to use his hands to play. *The Caring Person's Guide* has been designed specifically to help with the physical management of the patient and thus create a useful basis for further work.

What does this Guide Consist of?

This guide is divided into four parts:

Part 1   Physical Assessment

Part 2   Treatment

Part 3   Care Review

Part 4   Planning a System

Who is the Key Worker?

The key worker is the person whose job it is to make sure that this guide has been filled in correctly and that any recommendations are carried out. Since this guide is primarily for use in mental handicap hospitals, the key worker is most likely to be a nurse. The key worker should work in much the same way as a parent to ensure that the patient is well cared for and happy.

It is recommended that the key worker should work through those channels of communication and authority already in existence in her place of work. At the same time, it is recommended that the role of key worker should be respected by those in authority as one which encourages the care giver to take greater responsibility for her patient.

Who is the Co-worker?

The co-worker has a similar role to that of the key worker and it is her job to ensure that recommendations are carried out when the key worker is not present. In the hospital setting the co-worker is most likely to be a member of the opposite shift to the key worker.

Use of Terms

Throughout this guide, the person being assessed is taken to be male and is referred to as the 'patient' and the care giver is taken to be female. The decision to call the person being assessed the 'patient' was made after considerable thought and discussion. This term was felt to be the most appropriate, not because the authors adhere to the medical model of care, but because the term suggests the continuing need for treatment. The decision to refer to the patient as male and the care giver as female was made for purposes of simplicity and clarity. The illustrations are, however, based on real people of both sexes.

The Illustrations

Since the illustrations are derived from our work with and observation of real people, most of whom have not had the benefit of consistent treatment, the pictures also demonstrate problems of deformity and abnormality of movement. These illustrations are intended to give encouragement and ideas to those working with similar populations and are not intended as a model of perfection for treatment. Only by working through the guide with the help of your physiotherapist, and by seeking advice from others, can the best possible treatment be devised for your patient. None of the examples discussed or illustrated bears any relation to particular individuals.

Part One
Physical Assessment

'We (have) emphasised the importance of carrying out a detailed assessment of the needs of each individual resident: this applies with even greater force to the profoundly handicapped.'

Helping Mentally Handicapped People in Hospital: A Report to the Secretary of State for Social Services by the National Development Group for the Mentally Handicapped, DHSS 1978.

Introduction to Part One

HOW DO I COMPLETE THIS ASSESSMENT?

1. Read the description at the start of each section carefully.
2. Make full use of the forms to explain your findings or to mention any difficulties you have in carrying out the assessment.

   Don't worry if a comment looks silly when written down; remember that the more information you put on the forms the easier it will be when you go on to plan treatment.

   Some of the sections are easier to fill in if you can compare your patient's limbs with those of a normal person. Therefore it may be helpful to have another member of staff on hand to assist you.

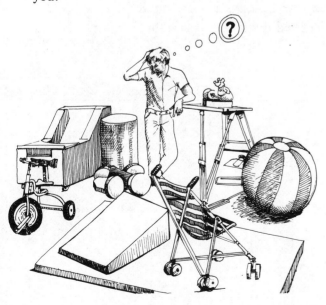

3. Remember to be sensitive to your patient's feelings and to talk to him as you work.
4. If you feel that your patient is in pain or is frightened, do not continue with that part of the assessment but try again on another day. If you get the same response when you try again, it is important not to try to pursue that area further but to make a note in the comments section of the reasons why that section has not been completed. Remember, this assessment is a means to an end—to help you to understand your patient's physical problems and to care for his needs in the best way possible.

WHAT EQUIPMENT DO I NEED?

You will need some equipment to do this assessment: a mat, a wedge, possibly a roll, a balance board and a special chair. It may be that during the assessment you will identify a need for special equipment, in which case make a note of it and mention it at the care review meeting. It can then be placed on the *shopping list*.

What does this Assessment Cover?

This physical assessment covers three main areas:

1. Muscle Tone
2. Deformity
3. Movement

These will be dealt with in separate sections. There are various diagrams, tables and illustrations to help you.

Assessment of Muscle Tone

Muscle tone is the state of readiness of muscles to contract. If you have normal muscle tone you are very lucky; your muscles work well together and are tight enough so that you do not fall to the floor and yet loose enough to allow you to move easily.

Your patient may have muscle tone which is generally too tight or too loose, or it may vary considerably.

HOW DO I FILL IN THIS SECTION?

This section consists of descriptions of muscle tone with a large stickman diagram. There is also a table to be filled in which will help you to identify general factors which affect your patient's muscle tone.

Decide which of the following descriptions applies to each of the limbs of your patient. The type of muscle tone should then be entered in the appropriate box on the diagram opposite. Perhaps the best way of deciding on the correct description of muscle tone is to ask another member of staff to help you. Try feeling her limbs when you move them and compare the ease with which they move with those of the disabled person.

Hypotonic

The limb feels heavy and floppy to move. If you feel across the muscles round the joint, they will be flabby. There may also be excess joint range, i.e., he may seem double-jointed.

Normal

The limb moves easily and smoothly in any direction that you indicate. The joint range should be normal as well.

Mild spasticity

The limb is slightly stiff and difficult to move. If you feel across the muscles round the joint they are slightly tight. There is a 'springiness' at the extremes of joint range so that the joint is reluctant to stretch or bend fully.

Moderate spasticity

The limb is difficult to move. If you feel across the muscles round the joint, they feel hard and stringy over some of the tendons. There may be some deformity of the joints. The patient may be sensitive and jumpy and tend to go into spasms. You will notice he tends to move in an odd, stereotyped way.

Severe spasticity

The limb is very stiff and difficult to move. The patient seems to be stuck in a few peculiar postures. The muscles feel hard and some of the tendons feel very prominent and stringy. There is likely to be deformity of the joints. If your patient is very spastic he will seem very jumpy and may react against sudden noises or rough handling with strong spasms.

Athetoid

When you try to move the limbs, they feel jumpy. When you move your hand across the muscles you can feel them twitching. When the patient tries to change position, he has uncontrollable movements.

Does your patient seem to be actively resisting movement? _____

In what position or positions did you place your patient in order to test muscle tone? _____

Does your patient's muscle tone seem to vary with:

		Comments
1.	Different positions	
2.	Emotion	
3.	Warmth	
4.	Cold	
5.	Medication	
6.	State of general health	
7.	Method of handling	
8.	Attempts to move	
9.	Other (please specify)	

Assessment of Muscle Tone

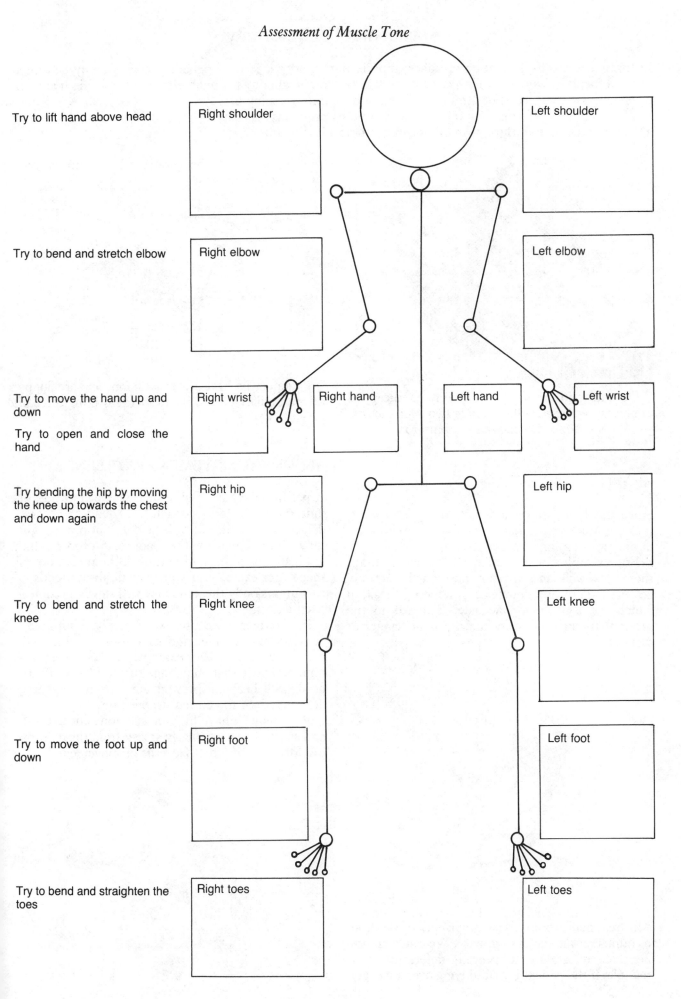

Try to lift hand above head

Try to bend and stretch elbow

Try to move the hand up and down

Try to open and close the hand

Try bending the hip by moving the knee up towards the chest and down again

Try to bend and stretch the knee

Try to move the foot up and down

Try to bend and straighten the toes

Right shoulder | Left shoulder
Right elbow | Left elbow
Right wrist | Right hand | Left hand | Left wrist
Right hip | Left hip
Right knee | Left knee
Right foot | Left foot
Right toes | Left toes

5

Assessment of Deformity

Deformity is the malformation of bones, muscles and tendons. If your patient becomes badly deformed many difficulties will arise: for example, he will become unable to sit, unable to move and his body will become so twisted that it will gradually destroy his ability to enjoy life.

Your patient's deformity can also cause enormous problems for those who look after him and he may appear unattractive to those who do not understand his difficulties.

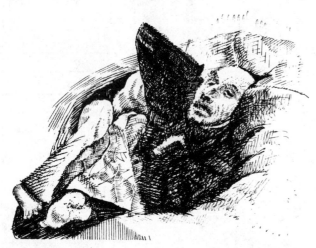

Deformity in the severely multiply handicapped can be caused by a combination of two main factors: **gravity** and **abnormal movement patterns**.

GRAVITY

Since gravity is a powerful force pulling downward, it can produce severe deformity if your patient stays in one position for long periods.

For example, many patients who cannot move their legs well and are not positioned correctly acquire a deformity known as 'wind-swept' legs, in which the legs lie to one side, flattened to the ground. In this deformity the hip is in danger of dislocating.

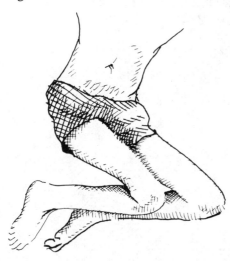

In treatment we use constant changes of position to counteract the forces of gravity. We can even use the force of gravity to prevent deformity. For example, if the patient is placed lying over a wedge,

the legs can then be positioned to help prevent 'wind-swept' deformity.

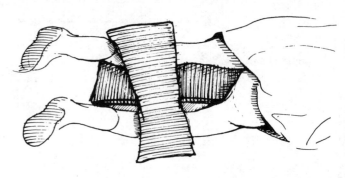

Patients who have low muscle tone and are floppy are particularly at risk from the deforming force of gravity.

ABNORMAL MOVEMENT PATTERNS

A person who has an abnormal way of moving, or indeed very little movement, will tend to become deformed over the years. If he does not bear weight through his bones they will not form properly and gradually his joints and bones will be pulled out of shape. For example, if your patient always tends to curl up his body this tendency will slowly become a fixed deformity.

In treatment, we use exercise, positioning and activities to encourage normal movement which will prevent deformity. For example, in the prone position, activities that encourage the patient to lift his head will help to prevent him from becoming deformed into the curled up position.

Patients who have high muscle tone and are stiff and spastic are particularly at risk from the deforming force of abnormal patterns of movement.

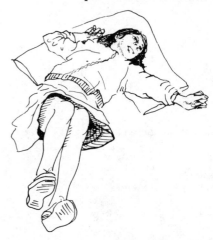

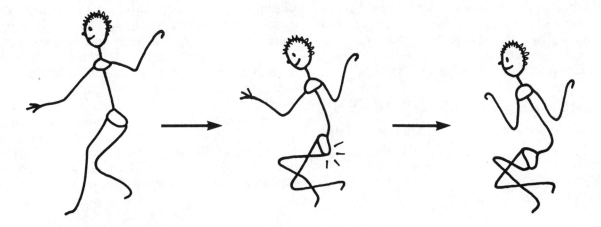

The child is lying on his back with his head usually turned to one side. The side to which the head is turned tends to stretch out and the other side tends to bend up (see ATNR, page 13).

The child's legs are lying to one side. The hip that is lying inwards dislocates. His arms and legs are tending to bend up and his trunk begins to bend sideways.

The patient's deformity gets worse. The trunk becomes very bent and the arms and legs are stuck in the bent position.

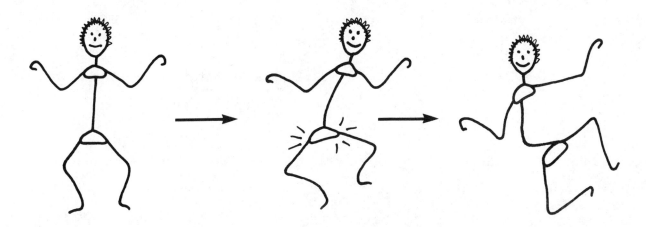

The child lies on his back. His legs flop out to each side.

The child's hips dislocate forwards making it impossible to bend him at the hips.

When attempts are made to put the patient in a sitting position, his spine bends.

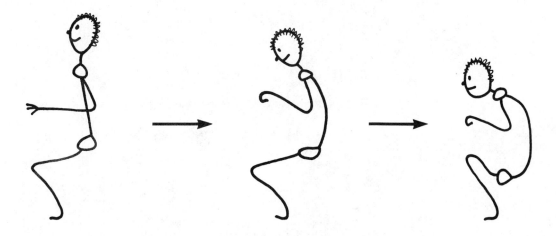

The child is able to be placed in a sitting position but cannot stand. He stays in the sitting position.

The child becomes hunched in sitting.

The patient's trunk and legs become so bent that he is no longer able to sit.

HOW DO I FILL IN THIS SECTION?

When filling in this section it is useful to enlist the help of another member of staff and compare her spine and limbs with those of your patient.

There are two subsections: the first deals with the *spine* and the second deals with the *limbs*.

How do I Tell if my Patient's Spine is Deformed?

There are three main types of deformity of the spine:
1. Scoliosis
2. Kyphosis
3. Lordosis

Opposite you will see simplified sketches of what each of these deformities looks like. Look at your patient from the front, behind and side, and try to draw in the boxes provided a sketch of the spine from each view. Then compare your sketch with those showing each type of deformity, decide whether there is a deformity and, if so, what it is.

Often, deformities of the spine are not as simple as the sketches opposite might suggest and therefore you may find it difficult to work out what the problem is. Draw the sketch as well as you can and ask the physiotherapist for help.

Assessment of Deformities of the Spine

Scoliosis (spine curves out sideways)

Concave to the left

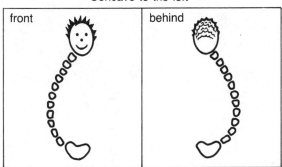

Concave to the right

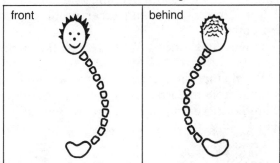

Kyphosis (hunched back)

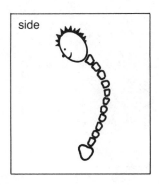

Lordosis of lumbar spine (bottom of spine affected: tummy bulges outwards)

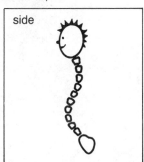

Lordosis of cervical spine (top of spine affected: chin pokes forward)

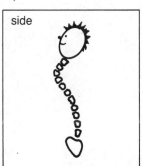

Your Patient

from front

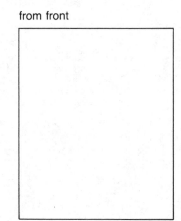

from behind

from side

How do I Tell if my Patient's Limbs are Deformed?

To identify problem areas, look at the diagram opposite and write in the appropriate box what you consider to be the condition of the joint; suggestions are listed, but if there are other problems write them down.

You may find it helps to try to draw the angle of the joints.

Note whether the deformity is severe or mild and if you are able to correct it or not (i.e., by moving the limb, can you make it look more normal?).

Assessment of Deformities of the Limbs

Shoulders
Normal
Hunched
Drawn back
Pushed forward
Pulled down

Elbows
Normal
Bent (flexed)
Straight (extended)

Wrists
Normal
Bent down (flexed)
Stretched back (extended)

Hands
Normal
Curled up
Stretched out
Thumbs across palm

Hips
Dislocated
Bent (flexed)
Straight (extended)
Crossed (abducted)
Normal
Turned in
Turned out

Knees
Bent (flexed)
Straight (extended)

Feet
Normal
Pointing down
Pulled up
Turned in
Turned out

Toes
Lifting up
Clawed

Right shoulder		Left shoulder
Right elbow		Left elbow
Right wrist	Right hand	Left hand	Left wrist
Right hip		Left hip
Right knee		Left knee
Right foot		Left foot
Right toes		Left toes

11

Assessment of Movement

The ability to move is important to us. We enjoy the ability to move and resent it when we have to stay still for a long time. We know that to remain in one position makes us stiff and uncomfortable. People who are severely multiply handicapped often have great difficulty in moving. They may find it difficult to move because of three main problems.

Problem 1

They may never have been encouraged to move and therefore find it strange and/or frightening, or they may have been discouraged and then lost interest in moving.

Problem 2

Their muscles may be too stiff, too floppy or too varied; that is, they have abnormal muscle tone.

A normal baby loses this reflex by the time he is about four to five months old but the baby with brain damage may find it much more difficult to lose this pattern of movement and may develop other bad movement habits. The cerebral palsied person finds it very difficult to lose these bad habits and often needs a lot of help.

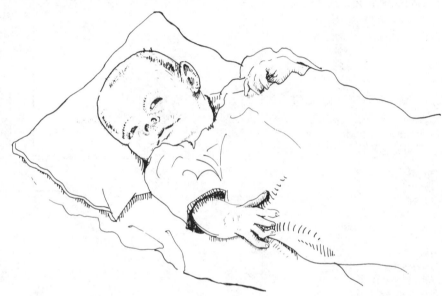

Problem 3

They may have bad patterns of movement. When a baby is born, he has certain patterns of movement. For instance, when he is about two months old he will have the reflex that whenever his face is turned to one side he will tend to stretch out the arm that he is facing and bend the other arm.

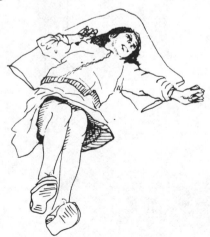

HOW CAN I TELL IF MY PATIENT HAS AN ABNORMAL PATTERN OF MOVEMENT?

Look carefully at the way your patient moves and feel for differences in muscle tone. For example, observe whether his arms and legs are affected by the position of his head. You may notice that his muscle tone changes when he is in different positions.

Described below are three abnormal patterns of movement which are fairly common in patients who suffer from cerebral palsy. They are called: *pathological tonic reflexes*. Your patient may show parts of these reflexes or he may have very abnormal patterns of movement which do not seem to fit these descriptions at all. It is often very difficult to tell which factors are affecting your patient's ability to move. The best guide to correct treatment is to think about what is normal in terms of movement and muscle tone and to aim to work towards that end. Try to keep these reflexes in mind when you are assessing how your patient moves.

Pathological Tonic Reflexes

Asymmetric Tonic Neck Reflex (ATNR)

If the patient's head is turned to one side, the side to which the head is turned tends to stretch out (i.e., is extended) and the other side tends to bend up.

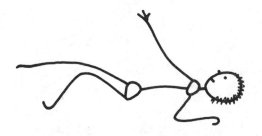

Symmetric Tonic Neck Reflex (STNR)

If the patient's chin is lifted, i.e., the head is extended, the arms will tend to stretch out and the legs bend up. If the chin is on the chest, i.e., the head is flexed, the arms may bend up and the legs tend to stretch out.

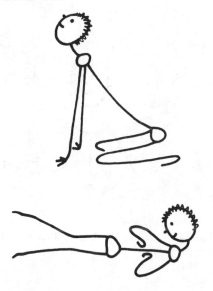

Tonic Labyrinthine Reflex

If the patient is lying on his back at an angle of 45° to horizontal, there is a generalised increase in extension, i.e., he becomes all stretched out.

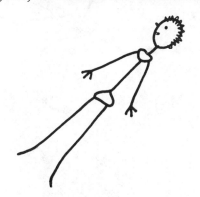

If the patient is lying on his front, with his head 45° below horizontal, there is a generalised increase in flexion, i.e., completely curled up.

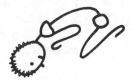

The prone position helps to overcome the effects of the tonic labyrinthine reflex.

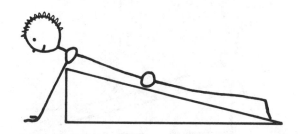

HOW DO I FILL IN THIS SECTION?

Throughout this section we shall consider the way a child learns to move. This is because we use normal development as a reference for comparison and guidance so that we can help those with movement difficulties to build up their abilities. The following tables have been devised to help you to look carefully at how your patient moves.

Fill in the boxes to show your patient's ability.

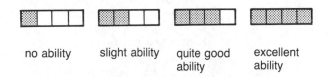

no ability   slight ability   quite good ability   excellent ability

Make Full Use of the Comments Column

Your patient may have different abilities on each side. Make a note in the comments column if this is so.

You may feel that there are sections of this assessment that do not apply to your patient:

- Some items may be much too difficult. Your patient may be too old, too young or have too many other problems for you to test his ability in this area. Don't give up too easily but write down the reasons why you believe an item may be too difficult.

- Some items may be much too easy, in which case make a note to this effect in the comments column.

Head Control

This is the cornerstone of all the posture and movement abilities. A patient needs to be able to control his head so that he can move, look and communicate. He needs to be able to control his head in order to chew and swallow properly. If he does not have head control he will remain essentially helpless.

Question

1. Can your patient be placed on his front? (Use a wedge if necessary.)

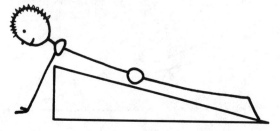

2. Can he lift his head while lying on his front?
3. Can your patient be raised up into a sitting position?

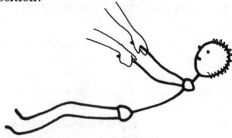

4. Can he lift his head as you raise him up into a sitting position?

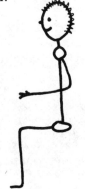

5. Can your patient be placed in a sitting position?

6. In sitting, can he:
   (a) control his head if you stabilise his shoulders?

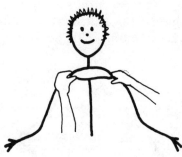

   (b) control his head if you stabilise his elbows?

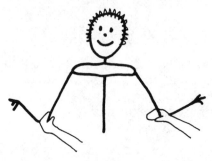

   (c) control his head if you stabilise his hands?

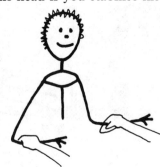

   (d) control his head if you lean him gently
       to the right?
       to the left?
       backwards?
       forwards?
   (e) move his head to look around?

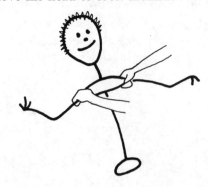

	No ability	Slight ability	Quite good ability	Excellent ability	Comments
1					
2					
3					
4					
5					
6a					
b					
c					
d					
e					
	No ability	Slight ability	Quite good ability	Excellent ability	Comments

Weight Bearing Through the Shoulders

This helps to make the shoulder girdle stable in order to give a firm foundation for the head and arms to work. The head and arms cannot work well if they are connected to wobbly shoulders.

Question

1. Can your patient be placed on his front?

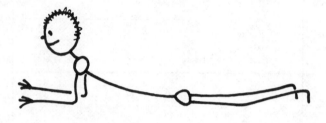

2. When on his front, can he:
(a) raise his head and shoulders and lean on his elbows?
(b) leaning on his elbows, move his head to look around?
(c) leaning on his elbows, reach with one hand, i.e., support himself on one elbow?

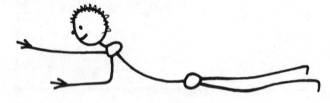

(d) raise his head and shoulders and lean on his hands with outstretched arms?

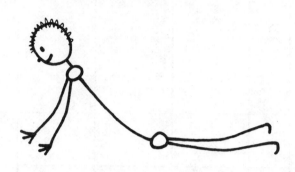

(e) on outstretched arms, move his head and shoulders to look around?
(f) on outstretched arms, move one hand and maintain his balance?

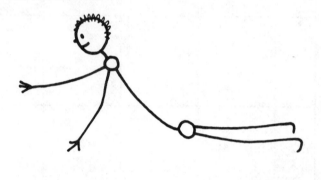

	No ability	Slight ability	Quite good ability	Excellent ability	Comments
1					
2a					
b					
c					
d					
e					
f					

Rolling

A baby quickly learns to roll from his front onto his back and later he learns to roll over and over. Some babies use this method to move around. Rolling is good for many patients, even if they need help. Remember, any movement is better than lying still. It can reduce spasticity and therefore help to prevent deformity.

Question

1. Can your patient roll from his front:
   (a) to his left side?
   (b) to his right side?
   (c) to his back?

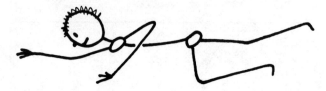

2. Can he roll from his back:
   (a) to his left side?
   (b) to his right side?
   (c) to his tummy?

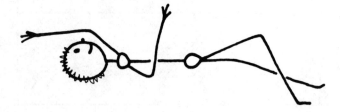

	No ability	Slight ability	Quite good ability	Excellent ability	Comments
1a					
b					
c					
2a					
b					
c					

Sitting

Babies first learn to sit by leaning on their hands in front of them. Slowly they learn to be more upright, to balance and then use their hands for other activities. Being able to balance in sitting without having to use the hands for support makes life much easier and makes activities such as independent feeding possible.

Question

1. Can your patient be placed in sitting?

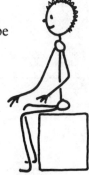

2. Can he raise his head in sitting:
   (a) with elbows stabilised at shoulder height?

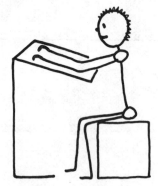

   (b) with elbows stabilised in front of him?

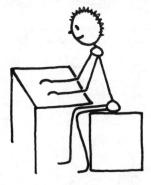

   (c) with hands stabilised in front of him?

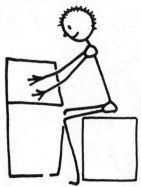

3. Can he reach with one hand while propping himself up with the other?

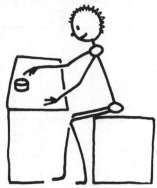

4. Can he put his hands down to prop himself up if you lean him gently:
   (a) to the front?

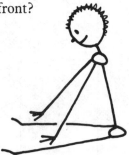

   (b) to the left-hand side?
   (c) to the right-hand side?

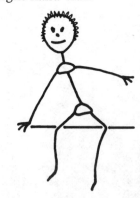

   (d) to the back?

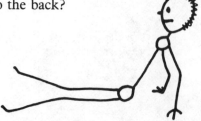

	No ability	Slight ability	Quite good ability	Excellent ability	Comments
1					
2a					
b					
c					
3					
4a					
b					
c					
d					

5. Can he balance without using his hands to prop himself up if you lean him gently:
   (a) to the front?

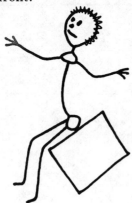

(d) to the back?

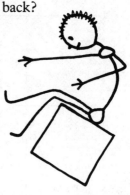

   (b) to the left-hand side?
   (c) to the right-hand side?

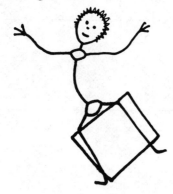

6. Can he balance in sitting and use both of his hands to reach out and play?

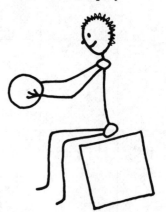

	No ability	Slight ability	Quite good ability	Excellent ability	Comments
5a					
b					
c					
d					
6					

Hand Function

Early in life a baby sees his hands and brings them together in front of him. He plays with them and brings them to his mouth. When he is beginning to sit, he learns to open them out and take weight on them for support. Gripping, patting, poking and waving have all got to be practised before he can go on to more complex actions. He watches his hands and practises using them for hours on end. Soon they become a useful tool. Your patient may be stuck at one of these stages, or perhaps he has never even seen his hands and does not know that they belong to him.

For this section you may find that your patient's ability to use his hands depends on his position. If his hands do not work well when he is lying on his back you will probably find that you can make it easier for him by one of the following ways: a good sitting position, side lying or on his stomach over a wedge. Experiment to find out the best possible position to help your patient use his hands and make a note in the comments column.

Question

1. Can he move his hand and fingers so as to feel different textures, e.g., own body and clothing?

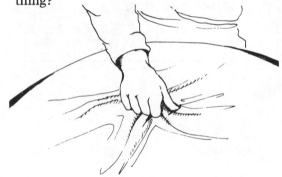

2. Can he take his hands to his mouth?

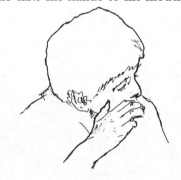

3. Can he grasp an object placed in the palm of his hand *and* release it at will?

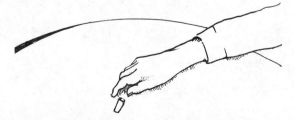

4. Can he reach out towards an object?

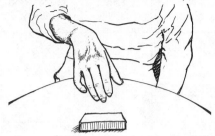

5. Can he take an object to his mouth?

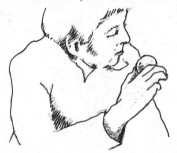

6. Can he take an object to his mouth and investigate what it is by tasting and shaking it?

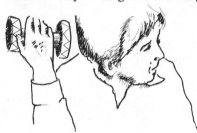

7. Can he take an object to his mouth and investigate what it is by shaking, tasting and looking at it?

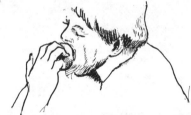

8. Can he transfer an object from one hand to another?

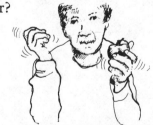

9. Can he pick up a cube (approximately 2.5 cm^3 of foam or wood) using the whole hand, i.e., can thumb and fingers rake the cube into the palm of his hand?

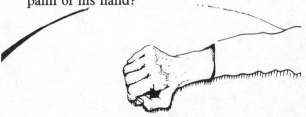

	No ability	Slight ability	Quite good ability	Excellent ability	Comments
1					
2					
3					
4					
5					
6					
7					
8					
9					

10. Can he pick up a cube using thumb against fingers?

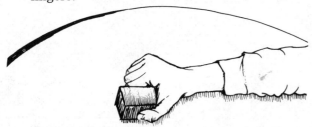

11. Can he pick up a cube using tips of thumb and fingers?

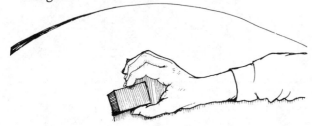

12. Can he pick up a pencil using the whole hand?

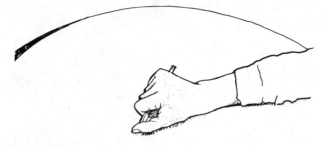

13. Can he pick up a pencil using thumb and fingers?

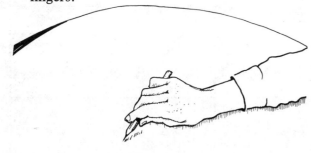

14. Can he pick up a pencil and:
(a) hold it to write in the normal way, i.e. using tips of thumb, index and middle fingers?
(b) move the pencil with fine control to draw small circles?

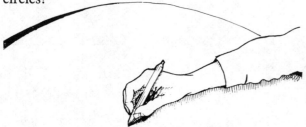

15. Can he pick up a Smartie using the whole hand, i.e. can his fingers rake the Smartie into the palm of his hand?

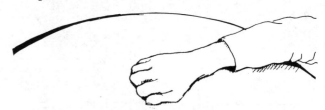

16. Can he pick up a Smartie using the thumb against curled index finger?

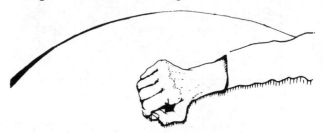

17. Can he pick up a Smartie using thumb and tip of index finger, i.e. in a pincer grasp?

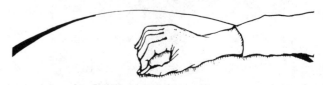

18. Can he pick up 'hundreds and thousands' using thumb and finger nail of index finger, i.e. a fine pincer grasp?

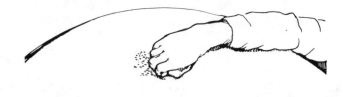

	No ability	Slight ability	Quite good ability	Excellent ability	Comments
10					
11					
12					
13					
14a					
b					
15					
16					
17					
18					

Use of Hands for Non-verbal Communication

If your patient is unable to speak it may be possible
for him to use his hands to help him communicate.
Makaton is a simple sign language which is often
used successfully by people who are severely multiply handicapped.

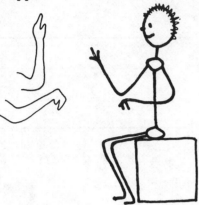

Question

1. Can he look at his hands?
2. Can he imitate simple signs, e.g. Makaton stage
   1, with a physical prompt?
3. Can he imitate simple signs without a physical
   prompt?
4. Can he use his hands in any consistent way to
   indicate need, e.g., gesturing? (Please specify
   all gestures used.)

	No ability	Slight ability	Quite good ability	Excellent ability	Comments
1					
2					
3					
4					

Weight Bearing Through Hands and Knees

This stage is the beginning of mobility. The patient who can move has an enormous advantage for learning and communicating. Weight bearing through hands and knees helps both the shoulders and hips to develop. Legs cannot work well if they are connected to wobbly hips. Hip joints develop well if they are used to bear weight and therefore they will be less likely to dislocate.

Question

1. Can your patient be placed on hands and knees?
2. Can he balance on hands and knees?

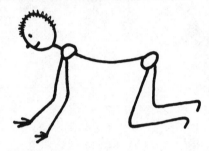

3. Can he balance on hands and knees when you push him gently:
   (a) forwards?
   (b) to the left?
   (c) to the right?
   (d) backwards?

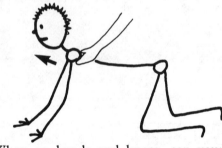

4. When on hands and knees, can your patient reach with one hand?

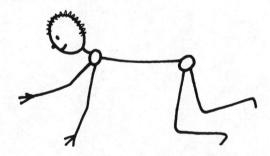

5. When on all fours, can he transfer weight from side to side?

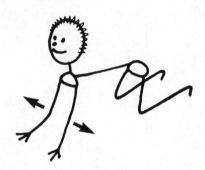

6. Can your patient crawl?

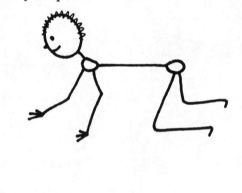

	No ability	Slight ability	Quite good ability	Excellent ability	Comments
1					
2					
3a					
b					
c					
d					
4					
5					
6					

Upright Kneeling

This is the next stage before standing. If your patient has wobbly hips and collapses when in standing, see if you can devise ways for him to practise upright kneeling.

Question

1. Can your patient be placed in upright kneeling with arms supported?
2. Can he balance in upright kneeling with arms supported?

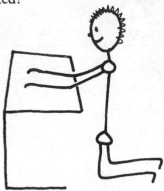

3. When in upright kneeling, can he reach with one arm?

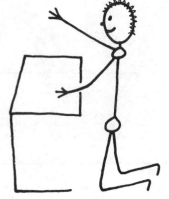

4. When in upright kneeling, can he balance with no arm support?

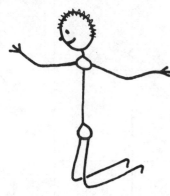

5. When in upright kneeling, can he reach and use his arms to play?

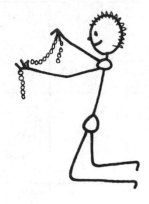

	No ability	Slight ability	Quite good ability	Excellent ability	Comments
1					
2					
3					
4					
5					

Standing

Standing can be very good for some patients; it encourages the formation of strong hip joints and helps to develop balance. Even if there is little hope of walking, standing with support is still recommended for many patients. There is a wide selection of different aids for standing. Ask the physiotherapist about these if you feel your patient might need this type of extra help.

Question

1. Can your patient be placed in standing with support? (In the Comments column please specify type of support needed.)

2. Can your patient take his weight in standing with support?

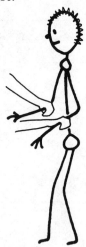

3. Can he transfer his weight from one leg to the other in standing with support?

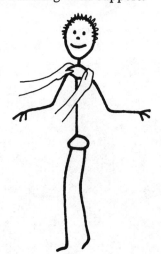

4. Can he pull himself up to standing with support?

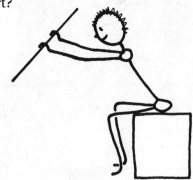

5. Can he step sideways with support?

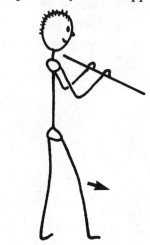

6. Can he stand without support?

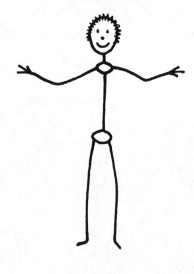

	No ability	Slight ability	Quite good ability	Excellent ability	Comments
1					
2					
3					
4					
5					
6					

Walking

Being able to walk is a very important skill. However, many people who are seriously disabled will never be able to walk. Even to take a few steps would be a great achievement.

Question

1. Can your patient stand with support? (Please specify type of support used.) _____

_____

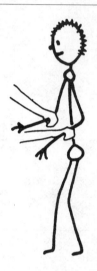

2. Can your patient stand with support and transfer his weight off his
   (a) right leg?
   (b) left leg?

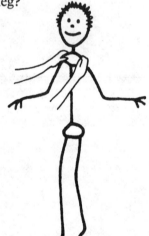

3. Can he lift his
   (a) right leg forwards?
   (b) left leg forwards?

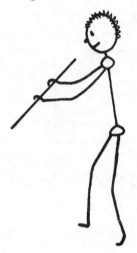

4. Can your patient walk a few steps with support?

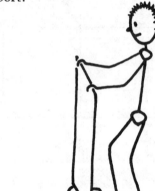

	No ability	Slight ability	Quite good ability	Excellent ability	Comments
1					
2a					
b					
3a					
b					
4					

Problems Page

What sort of *problems* are created *for your patient* by the inability to move well, abnormality of muscle tone or presence of deformity? For example, if his head is often dropped forward it may be difficult for him to see what is going on around him. If his fingers are often straight it may be almost impossible for him to hold objects such as a spoon, toys, etc.

In the care of your patient, what sort of *problems* are created *for you* by his inability to move well, abnormality of muscle tone or presence of deformity? For example, if his arms are bent it may make dressing difficult. If his hands are fisted this may create problems when cutting his nails. If his head is often thrown back, feeding may be a problem.

Anything that is a problem for your patient is likely to be a problem for you, too. Therefore, you are asked to write briefly about any such problems in the boxes provided.

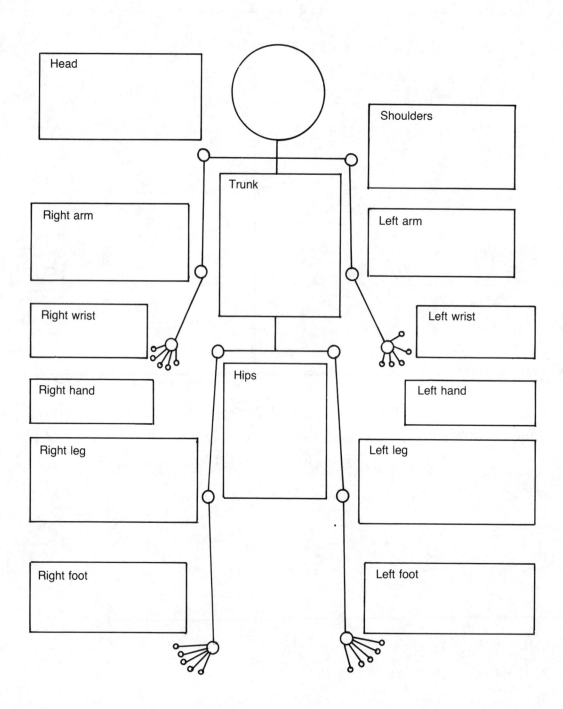

POSSIBLE FUTURE PROBLEMS

On the problems page you have written about the present problems of your patient and how they affect your job of caring for him. Imagine what would happen if these problems were left untreated and allowed to become worse.

A slight tendency to cross the legs may not pose practical problems when it is first noticed but if the legs are allowed to become fixed in the crossed position there may be problems with hip dislocation, toileting, pressure sores, sitting, etc.

Think carefully about what could happen to your patient if he is not treated but remember that despite the best possible treatment, some patients have such severe abnormality of movement that deformity is inevitable. If you have done all that is possible to prevent deformity, do not despair if you are not completely successful. Be encouraged by the knowledge that your patient would have been a lot worse if you had not worked hard with him.

Part Two

Treatment

'As to the therapy needed by physically handicapped children, it would be most helpful if this could be given by the staff who have most contact with the children, that is as a 24-hour 'way of life' for the children rather than as something that is 'done to' them for short periods on premises away from their wards.'

(Maureen Oswin (1978). *Children Living in Long Stay Hospitals*, Spastics International
Medical Publications, Research Monograph 5, Heinemann, London)

Introduction to Part Two

Now that you have identified some of the problems and needs of your patient, it is time to think about treatment. The following are some suggestions for treatment which are directed at:

● Solving some of the problems identified.

● Preventing deformity.

● Helping your patient to learn new skills.

This treatment is divided into four sections covering:

1. Positioning
2. Encouraging normal and active movement
3. Preventing deformity
4. Lifting and handling

At the end of each section you will be asked to think about whether the particular method described would be good for your patient, and to add any comments about how you might use the method.

Ask the doctor or physiotherapist if you are unsure about any of the suggested treatments.

Positioning

If a patient is very severely handicapped and cannot move very well, positioning is the main weapon to prevent deformity.

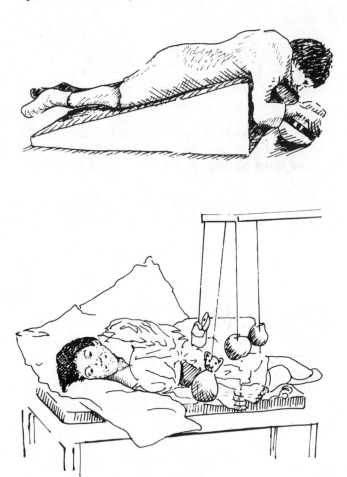

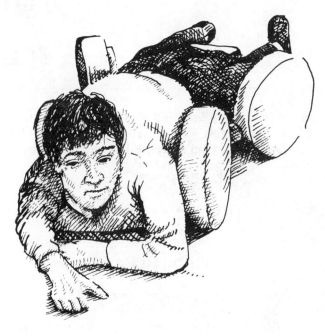

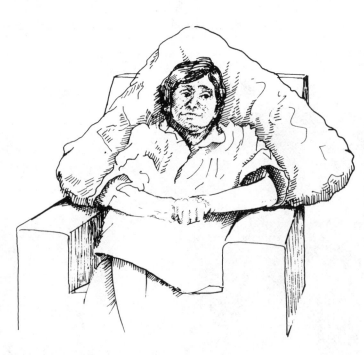

If your patient is kept moving from one position to another he is much less likely to become deformed.

Certain positions will be especially good for some patients and these positions will depend on their particular problems.

Normally we move about and change position frequently. We seldom stay still for any length of time except when necessary, e.g., on a long car journey. Remember what a relief it is to get out and stretch your legs.

Therefore, the aim should be twofold: to have at least two or three positions for each patient and to keep him moving throughout the day.

A list of equipment and aids to positioning, along with a summary of their uses, is given at the end of this section (page 47).

THE PRONE POSITION

This can be an extremely good position for the severely disabled person. *Why is it so good?*

- In the prone position the cerebral palsied person who is severely disabled may be less controlled by pathological reflex activity.

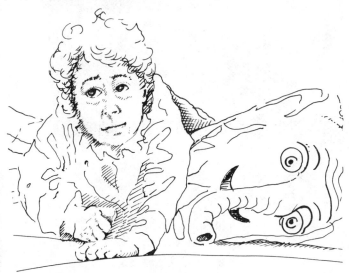

- In this position he is able to practise lifting his head and bearing weight on his elbows and hands.
- The prone position will help to prevent your patient from becoming deformed into a curled up position.
- It helps to straighten his back, hips and knees.
- It helps to prevent hip dislocation.

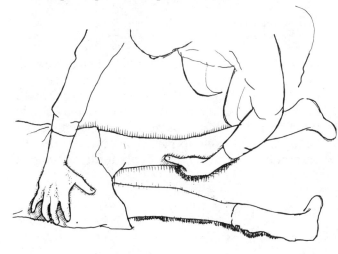

- Tummy trolleys can make it possible for some patients to move about in the prone position. This can encourage extension and can also be great fun.

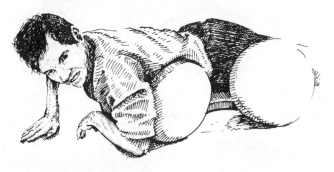

- The prone position is good for the patient who can walk but tends to bend his knees too much. In this case it helps to encourage him to stretch up and walk straight. For these patients the use of a tummy trolley is important so that their walking ability can be improved.

Do you think the prone position would be good for your patient? _____

If *yes*, does your patient need:

	Yes/no	If *yes*, specify type (if you need to order items please add to shopping list)
Wedge		
Sandbags		
Sheepskin		

Do you think that a tummy trolley would be a good idea for your patient? _____

If your patient can be placed on a tummy trolley but is unable to use his hands and arms to propel himself, do you think he could use an electric-powered tummy trolley? _____

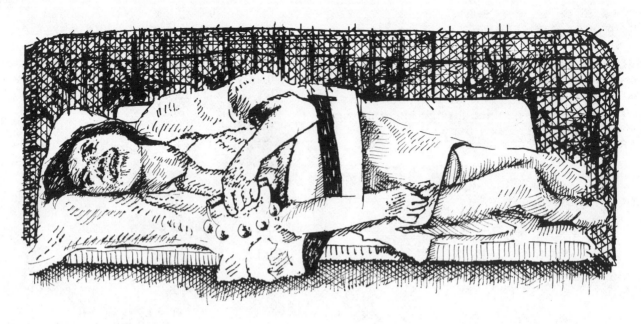

SIDE LYING

Side lying is useful because it stops the patient from pushing his head backwards and arching his back (extension). It also keeps the shoulders forward and allows the arms to come into the midline position. If your patient is affected by the asymmetric tonic neck reflex (ATNR, see page 13), side lying is useful since it helps to make the body more symmetrical.

Do you think side lying would be good for your patient? _____

If *yes*, does your patient need:

	Yes/no	If *yes*, specify type (if you need to order items please add to shopping list)
Side lying board		
Pummel		
Sandbags		
Sheepskins		

Note Some patients dislike side lying for two main reasons. It often requires them to be positioned on the floor where they cannot see or join in easily with activities around them and where there may also be more draughts. Try to arrange your patient so that he is warm and able to participate in activities, for example, by using a raised platform or adapted table.

44

SITTING

It is essential to provide a good sitting position for your patient in order to make it as easy as possible for him to use his hands. A good sitting position should also help to prevent deformity.

Try your patient in different chairs and experiment with supports. He may not be comfortable in a chair that is designed for you or me. Most people have an upright chair for mealtimes and a comfortable chair for relaxing. Your patient may need two or three different chairs, and the type required will depend on the activity he is performing. For example, a chair that is suitable for feeding may be intolerable if used for long periods of time.

Remember, a change of sitting position is good. *It is unacceptable to leave your patient in a wheelchair or in any one position for long periods.*

Think carefully about how a normal baby develops the ability to sit and ask the physiotherapist about how you can help your patient to acquire this important skill.

Can your patient be placed in a sitting position?

_____

If *no*, why not? _____

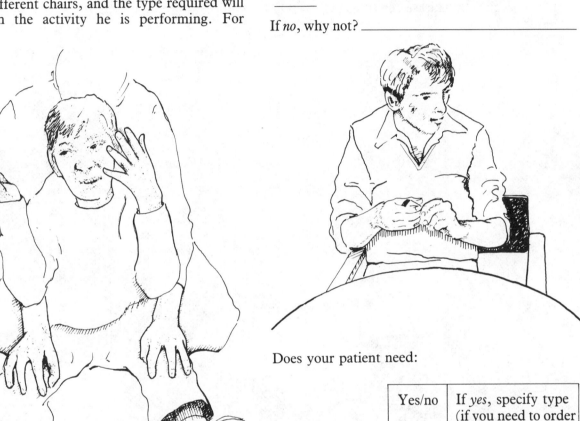

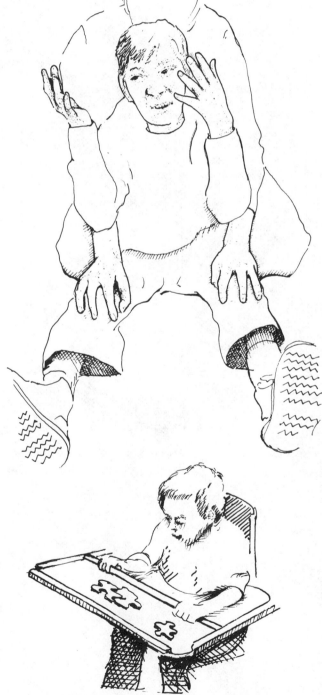

Does your patient need:

	Yes/no	If *yes*, specify type (if you need to order items please add to shopping list)
Special feeding seat		
Special armchair		
Special toilet seat		
Special car seat		
Wheelchair		
Wheelchair insert		
Sandbags		
Sheepskin		
Tri-pillow		

NIGHT-TIME POSITIONING

Corrective night-time positioning can be a very convenient and effective way of preventing deformity without too much disruption of your patient's daytime routine. You may need aids to help with positioning (see page 47) and/or aids to prevent deformity (see page 58).

What sleeping position(s) do you think would be best for your patient? (Please describe briefly.) ____

____

Does your patient need:

	Yes/no	If *yes*, specify type (if you need to order items please add to shopping list)
Sandbags		
Sheepskin		
Tri-pillow		
Night splints		

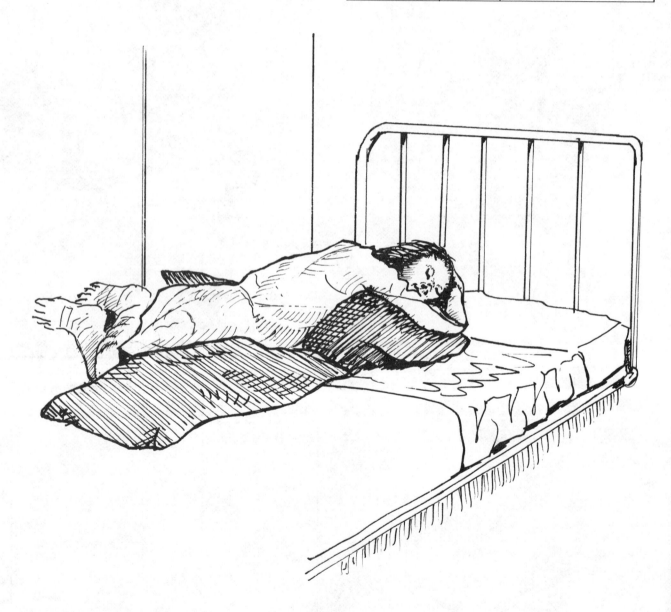

AIDS TO POSITIONING

Listed below are some items which may be necessary to help you position your patient.

EQUIPMENT	USES
Sandbags These should be of many different sizes. They can be home-made. Useful dimensions are 60 cm × 50 cm, 50 cm × 25 cm and 25 cm × 10 cm.	Sandbags are an invaluable and versatile aid to positioning. The weight provides a gentle but effective force which can be used to support and to restrict unwanted movement.
Sheepskins Washable artificial sheepskins are best since they allow for problems of incontinence.	Sheepskins provide comfort for those who cannot move easily. They reduce the risk of sores developing. Any form of discomfort will increase spasticity and therefore make the patient's condition worse.
Bolsters These can be made to your own specification to suit your patient's needs.	Bolsters can be used for prone lying, sitting or sitting astride to help develop balance.
Tri-pillows These are triangular-shaped pillows. It is often advisable to have a waterproof cover under the pillowcase.	A tri-pillow can provide comfort and support and can be used in a variety of ways to aid positioning. In the sitting position the pillow can be used to support the head and to bring the shoulders forward to support the arms, or perhaps to help position the legs. It is also useful in side lying and in lying prone.
Wedges The size of wedge and density of foam are important. Make sure that you have the right size for your patient and that the wedge is soft enough for comfort but firm enough for support.	Wedges can be used for prone lying, particularly when the patient is unable to bear weight through the shoulders for long periods.
Side lying boards These can be made straight or curved to provide a corrective position. A pummel or straps can be used to maintain the correct side lying position.	Side lying can be very beneficial since it can reduce extension and enable the patient to bring his hands together in midline. Some patients can use their hands better in side lying than in any other position.
Upright chairs These are often made from wood with some padding for comfort. They can have many adaptations to allow for correct positioning.	Upright chairs are used to encourage the development of balance in sitting. They would be uncomfortable and would therefore increase spasticity if used for long periods.
Armchairs These can be made out of foam to suit your patient's requirements. The gentle support of a chair made out of approved fire-resistant foam reduces spasticity and allows for correct and comfortable seating.	Special armchairs provide comfortable seating for times during the day when your patient needs to relax.
Tables These can be adapted in many ways to provide support in sitting or standing. Height and angle adjustments, along with cut-out sections, hand rails, elbow blocks and padding, can make this basic piece of equipment suitable for even the most severely handicapped.	Support in sitting or standing can be varied according to the patient's requirements.

Encouraging Normal and Active Movement

With skilled and specialised handling, and the correct equipment, you will be able to help your patient to control his movement in a way that may otherwise be impossible for him on his own. There are rules of handling that must be learnt and practised if you are to see the best results. Phy-siotherapists call this 'therapeutic handling'. Ask your patient's physiotherapist to help you with this section.

Look back to your movement assessment in Part One (pages 12 to 37) and check on the way you graded your patient's ability to move.

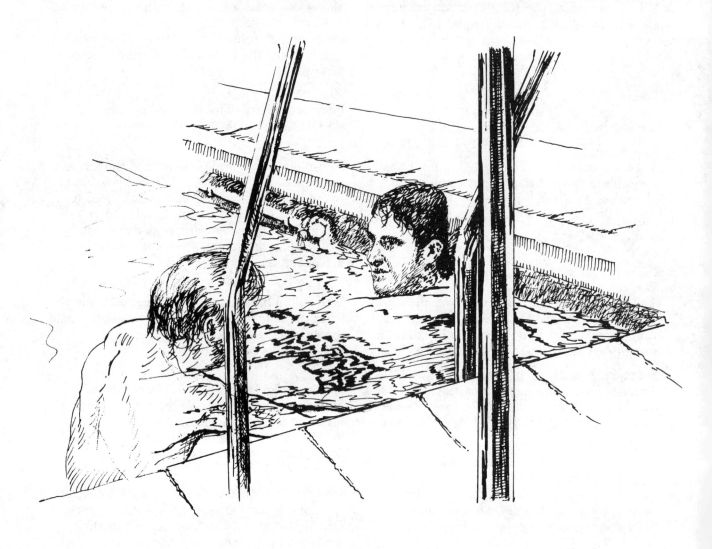

◻ **no ability**

Think carefully *why* your patient has no ability in a particular area. People who have very poor movement need to be positioned correctly to enable them to use the small amount of ability they have.

Your patient may be completely helpless if left lying on his back but he may have useful ability if positioned in side lying, sitting or on his front over a wedge.

If you think that your patient has no ability to clap his hands, ask yourself *why*. Is he in the best position? Does he know he has hands? Can he see his hands? Can he feel his hands? Can he bring them together? Can he open them?

Your patient must want to move but the effort of moving may be very great and many severely disabled people have lost ability because of lack of opportunity or encouragement, or increasing deformity.

Severely multiply handicapped people can often move in a way that surprises even those who know them well if the right opportunity and encouragement are given.

◻ **slight ability**

If your patient has slight ability at a particular skill, *this is the area that needs work*.

◻ **quite good ability**

If your patient has quite good ability at a particular skill, he will benefit from the opportunity to *practise*.

◻ **excellent ability**

If your patient is excellent at a particular skill, you should *move on* to more advanced activities.

People who are severely multiply handicapped sometimes have little opportunity to discover new activities and there is always a danger that they may become obsessed with repeating a skill over and over again. For example, some patients find it difficult to *move on* from the fascination of bringing their hands to their mouth. If your patient is stuck with one activity, you will need help to learn how to encourage him to try something new.

To Summarise

| No ability ◻ | Ask yourself *WHY NOT?* | Quite good ability ◻ | *PRACTICE* will be worthwhile |
| Slight ability ◻ | *WORK* needed | Excellent ability ◻ | *MOVE ON* to more advanced activities |

Head Control

Does your patient need *work* or *practice* to help him to develop head control? _____

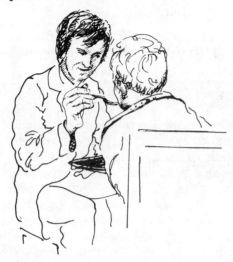

If *yes*, what activities can you think of to help him to practise head control? _____

_____

_____

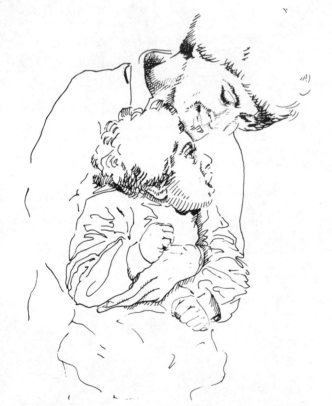

What equipment do you need for these activities?

_____

_____

Weight Bearing Through the Shoulders

Does your patient need *work* or *practice* to help him to develop weight bearing through the shoulders?

_____

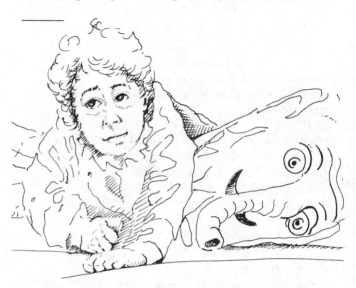

If *yes*, what activities can you think of to help him to practise weight bearing through the shoulders?

_____

_____

_____

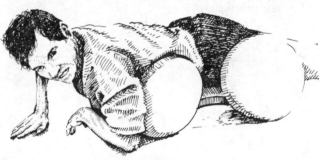

What equipment do you need for these activities?

_____

_____

_____

Rolling

Does your patient need *work* or *practice* to help him to develop the ability to roll? _____

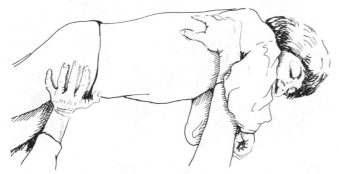

If *yes*, what activities can you think of to help him to practise rolling? _____
_____
_____

What equipment do you need for these activities?
_____
_____
_____

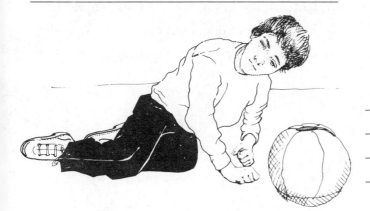

Sitting

Does your patient need *work* or *practice* to help him to sit? _____

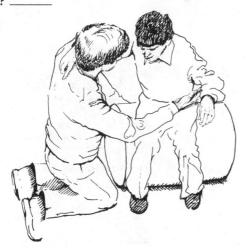

If *yes*, what activities can you think of to help him to practise sitting? _____
_____
_____

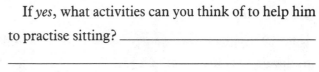

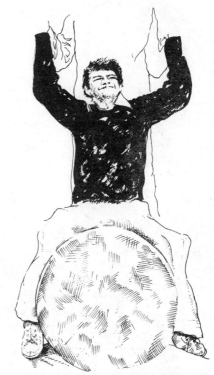

What equipment do you need for these activities?
_____
_____
_____
_____

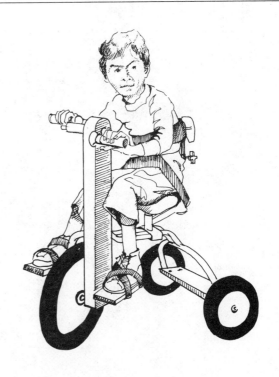

Hand Control

Does your patient need *work* or *practice* to help him to develop hand control? _____

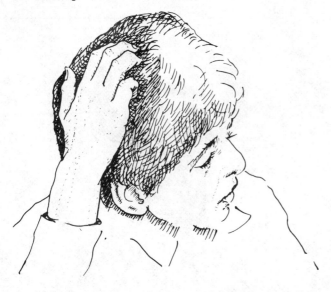

If *yes*, what activities can you think of to help him to practise hand control? _____

_____

_____

_____

_____

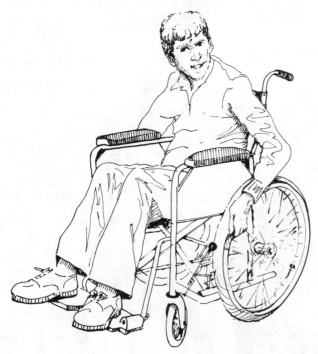

What equipment do you need for these activities?

_____

_____

_____

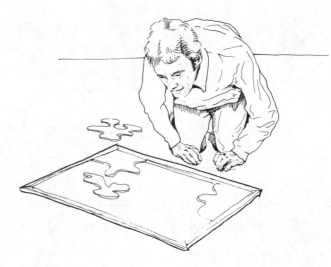

Weight Bearing Through Hands and Knees

Does your patient need *work* or *practice* to help him to develop weight bearing through hands and knees? _____

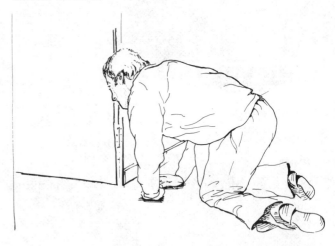

If *yes*, what activities can you think of to help him to practise weight bearing through hands and knees?

_____

_____

_____

What equipment do you need for these activities?

_____

_____

_____

Upright Kneeling

Does your patient need *work* or *practice* to help him to develop upright kneeling? _____

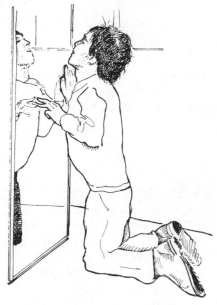

If *yes*, what activities can you think of to help him to practise upright kneeling? _____

_____

_____

What equipment do you need for these activities?

_____

_____

_____

Standing

Does your patient need *work* or *practice* to help him to develop the ability to stand? _____

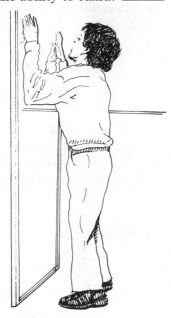

If *yes*, what activities can you think of to help him to practise standing? _____

_____

_____

What equipment do you need for these activities?

_____

_____

_____

Walking

Does your patient need *work* or *practice* to help him to develop the ability to walk? _____

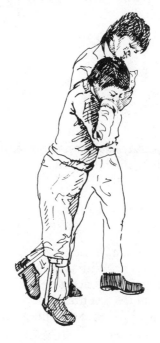

If *yes*, what activities can you think of to help him to practise walking? _____

_____

_____

What equipment do you need for these activities?

_____

_____

_____

_____

AIDS TO ENCOURAGE NORMAL AND ACTIVE MOVEMENT

There are many specialised aids to help you to encourage normal and active movement. Everyday objects can also be invaluable if used with imagination.

Listed below are a few examples of specialised and non-specialised equipment with a brief description of possible benefits.

EQUIPMENT	BENEFITS
Standing frames Many different types are available. They can provide upright support or can be inclined for the less able patient. They can be handmade out of wood or selected from a wide range of commercially available standing frames.	Standing frames provide support for those who cannot stand alone. Standing can be very beneficial in developing balance and in encouraging weight bearing.
Walking aids These range from a simple walking stick to aids which provide a large degree of support for the body.	These can be used to provide support and protection when walking and are suitable for patients who (1) have the ability to bear weight in standing, (2) are able to transfer weight from one leg to the other and (3) are able to take some steps. There is no therapy in supporting a patient in a walking aid if he does not have some ability in weight bearing and balance.
Adapted tricycles Even quite severely handicapped patients can benefit from tricycling if the equipment is adapted to suit them.	Tricycling can be excellent therapy and great fun. Amongst other benefits, it can help to strengthen legs, improve balance, encourage head control and body symmetry.
Wheelchairs The wheelchair must be the right size and shape for the patient. With adaptations (whether standard or home-made) the wheelchair can be made to accommodate and correct many problems. For some patients a wheelchair insert may be necessary. There is a very wide range of commercially available wheelchairs and there are different models of wheelchair for different purposes. *Note* The DHSS will supply a wheelchair for your patient. If he needs the sort of wheelchair that does not fold, the DHSS will also supply a wheelchair that folds for transit purposes.	Many obvious benefits are achieved by the increased mobility provided by wheelchairs. Every patient should be able to benefit from a wheelchair although some may need special adaptations. The most severely deformed patients may need a wheelchair insert to enable them to use the equipment without discomfort. If you think that your patient could use his hands and arms to propel himself, make sure that the wheelchair has big wheels which he can reach.
Electric wheelchairs and trolleys These can be adapted so that even a small amount of controlled movement in any part of the body can be used to operate the vehicle.	These can encourage purposeful movement and can give independence to some patients. Even if the patient always needs supervision it can be a unique and exciting experience for a severely multiply handicapped patient to move independently.

EQUIPMENT	BENEFITS
Hydrotherapy pools, Jacuzzis, paddling pools and baths Many schools and institutions for the disabled have a hydrotherapy pool which is usually kept at a warm temperature. Jacuzzi baths provide buoyancy and a massaging effect. Paddling pools, indoor or outdoor, can also be used to provide hydrotherapy. An ordinary bath can be used to provide regular hydrotherapy.	The facility to move about in water can be of great value to the severely handicapped. Often a patient is able to move in water in a way which is impossible on dry land. Spasticity can be reduced by the warmth and movement of water.
Adapted saddles for horse riding There are many commercially available saddles for the disabled.	Horse riding can help to develop balance in sitting. It can help to reduce spasticity in the legs and can provide an ideal opportunity to look down on the world instead of always being looked down upon! *Note* Even if your patient is too handicapped to ride a horse he may enjoy a ride in a horse-drawn carriage.
Tummy trolleys These are commercially available or can be home-made. The size and shape of the tummy trolley should be chosen carefully to suit the needs of the patient.	Tummy trolleys can be invaluable to provide mobility and exercise. Use of a tummy trolley encourages extension and strengthens the arms, wrists and shoulders.
Play equipment and adapted toys A great many commercially available items of play equipment can be used (with or without adaptation) to encourage normal and active movement. Items can be home-made and sometimes a toy maker or handyman can design and make a special toy for you. Toys which produce a large response for only a small amount of effort are best. Battery operated toys can be converted so that they can be operated by even the most severely handicapped. Mobiles, mobile stands, adjustable tables, G clamps and non-stick mats are also invaluable items.	The benefits of using toys and play to encourage your patient to move are almost limitless. If your patient is relaxed and enjoying himself, the results of this therapy are likely to be more rewarding for him and you.
Vibration Equipment which produces mechanical vibration specifically for medical purposes is commercially available.	The use of vibration for treatment is a relatively new technique. It is claimed to be useful for influencing muscle tone, aiding circulation, helping to reduce lung congestion and for providing a source of enjoyment.

Preventing Deformity

Preventing deformity is an essential part of the nursing care of the severely disabled patient.

If every effort is made to prevent deformity, your patient should be able to use conventional wheelchairs, furniture, etc.

If your patient is allowed to become severely deformed, the resulting problems may destroy his quality of life and make life very difficult for those whose job it is to look after him.

Various aids can be used to break up spastic patterns of movement. If feet and hands are kept straight it helps the whole body to move well.

Thoughtful use of aids can help to make sure that your patient does not suffer the appalling discomfort of severe deformity.

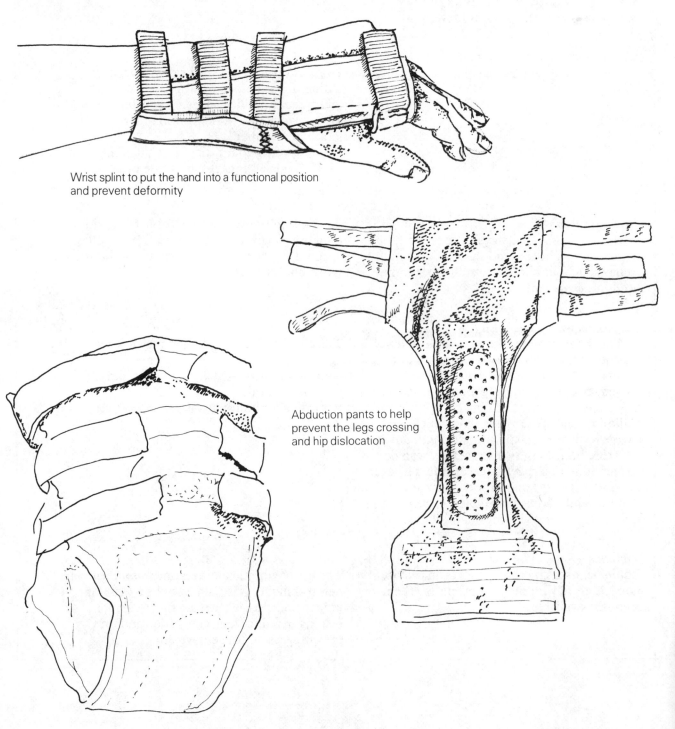

Wrist splint to put the hand into a functional position and prevent deformity

Abduction pants to help prevent the legs crossing and hip dislocation

If you think that your patient needs aids to prevent deformity please ask his physiotherapist and doctor for more information and advice, since many of the aids to prevent deformity require a prescription and skilled fitting. A list of equipment and aids to help prevent deformity is given on page 58.

Does your patient need:

	Yes/no	If *yes*, please specify type (if you need to order any items please add to shopping list)
Boots and shoes		
Body brace		
Splints		
Abduction pants		
Leg gaiters		
Arm gaiters		
Serial plasters		
Splintage for toes		

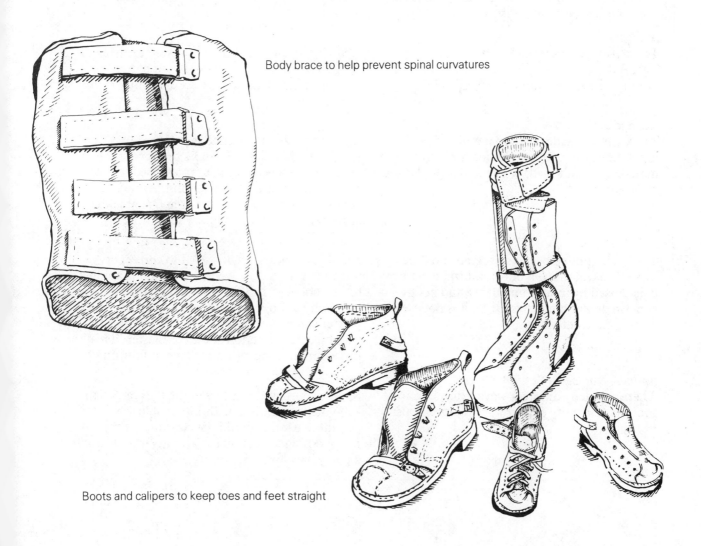

Body brace to help prevent spinal curvatures

Boots and calipers to keep toes and feet straight

AIDS TO PREVENT DEFORMITY

EQUIPMENT	USES
Boots and shoes Many different types of boots and shoes are available either from a standard range or made to measure.	Boots and shoes are used to prevent the feet from becoming deformed. They should be used consistently throughout the day in order to be effective. Those who cannot walk, run the risk of developing deformity of the feet and, therefore, even if a patient is unable to walk, correct footwear should be an indispensable part of his wardrobe.
Calipers These are made individually to a doctor's prescription.	Calipers can be used when the support of a boot or shoe is not sufficient.
Body braces These are also made individually to a doctor's prescription. There are many different types of body brace and they can be made from many different materials, therefore they need specialist manufacture and fitting.	Body braces are used to prevent the development of deformities of the spine. They have to be used consistently in order to be effective.
Splints These can be made from many different types of materials. Some are commercially available and some are made to measure.	Splints can be used for support, to prevent unwanted movement and to prevent deformity.
Abduction pants These pants provide thick padding between the legs. A double nappy pinned at both sides can produce the same effect on a smaller child.	Abduction pants are used to prevent crossing of the legs from becoming a dominant pattern of movement and thus to prevent deformity from developing.
Leg and arm gaiters These can be made out of material with stiffening, plastazote (a supportive foam which can be moulded when heated) or even thick, rolled-up newspaper.	Arms and legs can be encouraged to stay straight with the use of gaiters to support the knees and elbows. Leg gaiters are used to support the knees when standing. Arm gaiters are used to stabilise the elbows and enable the arms to be used for support when sitting.
Serial plasters These are applied by physiotherapist or doctors. This technique is only used when deformity is caused by muscle imbalance and not by abnormality of bone shape, i.e., it is not used to correct fixed deformity.	Serial plasters are usually used to correct deformity of the feet or wrists. A plaster is applied to the foot or wrist with as much correction of deformity as possible. After about ten days the plaster is removed and it is usually possible to gain further correction and to re-plaster. This procedure may be repeated three or four times.
Splintage for toes There are many different ways to use tape to prevent deformity of the toes. Splints can also be used.	Simple splintage or taping of the toes can often keep the toes straight and thus enable the patient to use standard boots or shoes. This method is only suitable for patients who do not already have fixed deformity.

Lifting and Handling

LIFTING AND CARRYING

There are many methods of lifting and carrying. It is important that your patient is lifted in a way that encourages him to control his own body and helps to prevent deformity. Two examples are given below.

For the Patient who Tends to Extend

For the Patient who Tends to Flex

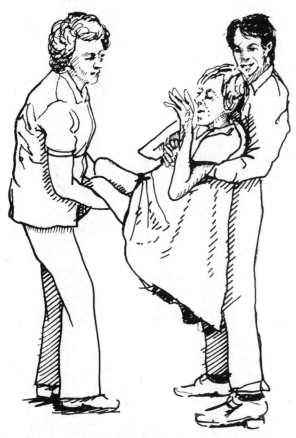

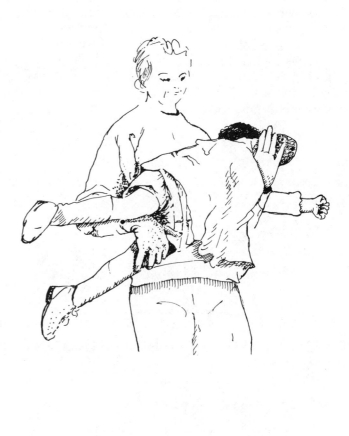

These two examples illustrate that it is important to use methods of lifting and carrying that reduce spasticity and help to correct abnormality of movement.

The methods of lifting and carrying your patient must be chosen carefully. Your patient may be big and heavy and/or have established strong abnormal movement patterns and/or severe deformity. Find out about the many different methods of lifting and carrying and which aids might be available.

Do you need more than one person to lift your patient? _____

Does your patient have abnormality of movement patterns which affect lifting? _____

Does your patient have severe deformity which affects lifting? _____

How do you think your patient should be lifted? (Describe methods briefly.) _____
_____
_____
_____

HANDLING

Methods of handling can have profound physical effects on the patient. Many patients develop marked increase in muscle tone and abnormality of movement in response to incorrect handling. Methods of handling should be chosen specially to suit the patient.

There are often 'tricks of the trade' which can make handling much easier for you and more beneficial for your patient. For example, for patients whose legs tend to become stiff, stretched out and crossed (extended and abducted) the process of nappy changing can become a form of treatment if the legs are bent and encouraged to part (flexed and abducted). This technique, if used regularly, will not only be good for the patient but will also make nappy changing easier.

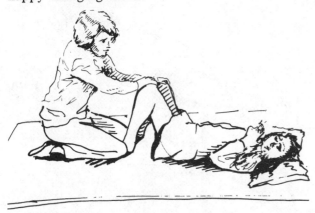

Find out about special methods of handling for your patient.

What special methods of handling do you think would be good for your patient? _____
_____
_____
_____

Correcting the tendency for the wrist to bend and the fingers to curl up.

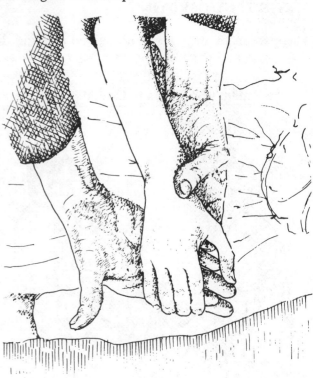

This leg tends to turn in and so needs special handling to turn it outwards as part of the treatment to prevent hip dislocation.

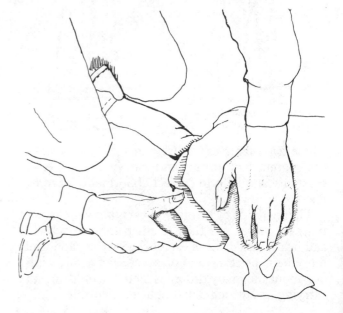

60

Part Three

Care Review

Introduction to Part Three

You have now assessed your patient and have some idea of what treatments might benefit him. The next step is to discuss your findings with all those involved with him. The care review meeting gives everyone the opportunity to put forward their suggestions, learn from each other and to agree a thorough and practical plan for his care.

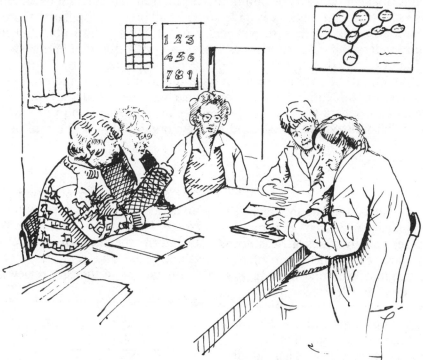

HOW DO I PRESENT ALL THE INFORMATION ABOUT MY PATIENT?

To help you in your job of presenting your patient to others at the care review meeting, and to ensure that all the information you have found is discussed, it is suggested that you make brief notes under the headings set out below.

Summary of Assessment Section

Problems identified (refer to pages 38 to 39)

Abilities identified (refer to Movement Section pages 14 to 37)

Summary of Treatment Section

Positioning (refer to pages 43 to 46)

Encouraging normal and active movement (refer to pages 50 to 53)

Preventing deformity (refer to page 57)

Lifting and handling (refer to pages 59 to 60)

The Care Review

This guide recommends that it should be the key worker's responsibility to organise the care review. However, as mentioned earlier, the key worker should work through all those channels of authority and communication already in existence in her place of work and should seek advice and support as necessary.

The aims of the care review should be twofold:

- The sharing of information about the needs and physical problems of the patient with everyone involved in his care.

- Discussion on what can be done to deal with the problems identified and to find out how the complex needs of the patient may be met.

Your patient should be present at the care review because it is an ideal opportunity to demonstrate specific treatment techniques and to explain the reasons why treatment is necessary. If this situation is handled with tact, it can be a very enjoyable occasion for him to be the centre of attention among interested and caring people.

As the multiply handicapped are a very difficult population with which to work, and since no one person or profession can have all the answers, it is vital that everyone present feels that their contribution, however small, is valued and valuable. It should be recognised that the use of jargon sometimes prevents people from understanding information about the patient's problems and possible solutions to them. Those who use jargon should therefore make it their responsibility to use practical demonstrations, along with explanations in lay terms, to make sure that their message is understood by all present. Similarly, those present at the care review meeting should also make it their responsibility to ask for a point to be explained again or made clearer if they do not understand. It is sometimes useful to have a question and answer format, whereby those who have the most knowledge of working with the patient ask each other questions to clarify points which other people present at the meeting may not have the confidence or the experience to ask.

Although it is important to identify problems and what will happen if they are not treated, it is also important to create an atmosphere sensitive to the feelings of the patient and those who care for him.

The general points that follow have been found to make organisation of the care review easier.

Timing

The first care review (that is, the one in which the findings of the guide are discussed and recommendations are made) usually takes at least two hours. (Subsequent care reviews need not take so long.) It is important that everyone attending is prepared for a meeting of this length.

It is also important to time the care review so that it falls during the least hectic part of the day; this may be particularly relevant if the meeting is taking place on a hospital ward. It may also be a good idea to make arrangements for someone to cover the ward so that as many staff as possible can relax and participate in the meeting.

The best time for the care review would be .... am/pm.

Attendance

The personnel who attend the care review meeting will depend on the setting in which you work. There are many people who should be able to contribute but it is worth while thinking carefully about who should be invited. Look back to the information sheet at the front of the guide to make sure that all those involved in your patient's care are invited.

Note Don't forget to involve your co-worker and to inform the medical officer that the meeting is taking place.

Invitations to the care review should be sent to:

_____

_____

_____

_____

_____

Structure

Although the care review should be as relaxed and informal as possible, it is also important that it is structured so that all the information is covered and that recommendations are discussed systematically. It is therefore essential to have an agenda. The following agenda has been found to cover the main points that are felt to be important and to provide a logical structure.

SUGGESTED AGENDA	ALTERNATIVE AGENDA

1. Introductions and apologies
2. Problems identified by key worker
3. Comments from others
4. Abilities identified by key worker
5. Comments from others
6. Discussion of treatments
  (including equipment needed and how to carry
  out recommended treatments)
  (a) Positioning
  (b) Encouraging normal and active movement
  (c) Aids to prevent deformity
  (d) Lifting and carrying
7. Summary of findings and recommendations
8. Date and time of next meeting to discuss progress
  with recommendations	

Do you think that this agenda will be of use for your care review? _____

If *no*, plan an alternative agenda in the space provided.

Note It might be a good idea to start the meeting with refreshments, since this often helps to create the right atmosphere for discussion.

Demonstrations

As mentioned earlier, the use of jargon should be avoided and wherever possible a point should be demonstrated.

The following are to be demonstrated at care review meetings:

_____

_____

_____

_____

_____

Equipment

Wherever and whenever possible all the equipment which you use with your patient should be assembled in the room where the care review is taking place so that the practical demonstrations can be carried out easily.

Don't forget to use the 'shopping list' and to bring catalogues, books and leaflets showing the equipment you may need to order.

Equipment needed for care review:

_____

_____

_____

_____

Note Taking

Notes should be taken throughout the care review and it is helpful if the person taking the notes stops the meeting periodically to sum up what has been said and to confirm that all present agree with what has been noted.

The note taker can be anyone who is prepared to take responsibility for the job of writing up and distributing the notes of the care review. However, it is recommended that the key worker should *not* be the person responsible for taking the notes.

For the purposes of clarity, it is a good idea to use the points of the agenda as subheadings when writing the notes up after the meeting. The key worker, physiotherapist and note taker should collaborate if necessary to make sure that the notes of the meeting are clear and accurate prior to their distribution.

The person responsible for taking the notes will be:

_____

Part Four
Planning a System

Introduction to Part Four

You have now held the *Care Review* and will know what has been recommended and agreed by all those present at the meeting. It is now necessary to make sure that these recommendations are carried out correctly, consistently and with continuity.

It is essential, therefore, to *plan a system* which ensures that everyone involved with your patient knows what has been recommended and how to carry out these recommendations reliably and regularly; that is, you need to decide how to *implement* the recommendations. In addition, it is necessary to know how you are going to find out if the recommendations are working and proving to be of benefit to your patient; that is, you need to plan a way in which you can *evaluate* the work carried out.

These two areas of *implementation* and *evaluation* tend to overlap and one cannot be planned without taking the other into account. However, for the purposes of simplicity and clarity they will be considered separately.

In order to plan a system which has every chance of being successful, you will need the support of many other people who are both directly and indirectly involved in your patient's care. For example, if the recommendations are to be implemented and evaluated in a hospital, it may be necessary to inform and consult people other than those responsible for the ward. For example: you may need to introduce equipment which will affect cleaning work; you may want to fix noticeboards to the wall which will involve work from another department; you may need to raise money for aids and activities. It is therefore important to think carefully about the setting in which you work and who should be consulted and informed.

Implementation

Think about how you are going to make sure that the recommendations agreed at the care review are carried out correctly, consistently and with continuity.

IDEAS FOR IMPLEMENTATION

Correctly

It is obvious that treatment will not be effective unless it is carried out in the correct manner; in fact you may do more harm than good.

Consistently

However correctly you carry out the treatment, it will be ineffective if it is not carried out consistently.

With Continuity

You must plan for a time in the future when you may no longer be able to be key worker for your patient. Therefore, it is necessary to make sure that all the information you have gained is not lost and that recommended treatments are continued.

IDEAS FOR IMPLEMENTATION

The following are some ideas which may be helpful with implementation; decide which methods you are going to use or think up some ideas of your own.

Demonstrations

Many treatments and methods of handling are difficult to describe in words. The key worker and physiotherapist can demonstrate to all involved how to carry out treatments and the best ways to handle the patient.

Will you use demonstrations to explain treatments?

_____

If *yes*, whom will you demonstrate to? _____

_____

What treatments and methods will you demonstrate?

_____

_____

Photographs

These provide an excellent visual record for reference. Explanations may be needed to accompany photographs.

Will you use photographs? _____
If *yes*, what recommendations will you photograph?

_____

_____

_____

Videos

Many institutions and private homes have their own video equipment and it may be possible to make a short film to show how to carry out the recommendations. This method has the advantage over photographs because it is easier to show techniques of handling and your patient's quality of movement. The tape can also be slowed down or frozen to illustrate a technique in more detail.

Will you use video? _____

If *yes*, what recommendations will you film? _____

_____

_____

_____

Diagrams and Notes

Some treatment principles are best explained by the use of diagrams and notes.

Will you use diagrams and notes? _____
If *yes*, what principles will you illustrate in this way?

_____

_____

_____

_____

Timetables and Checklists

Timetables and checklists can be helpful as reminders to you and others about how and when recommendations should be carried out. They are particularly useful for those who have more than one patient to care for.

Will you use timetables/checklists? _____

If *yes*, what information will these timetables and checklists contain? _____

_____

_____

Wall Charts

A visual display can be useful in a busy environment such as a hospital ward. Displays may include photographs, timetables, diagrams and anything which could be of use to those caring for your patient. For example, night-time positioning charts showing the use of splints and sleeping positions to prevent deformity can be used to involve night staff in the active treatment of your patient.

Will you use wall charts? _____

If *yes*, what information will be displayed? _____

_____

_____

_____

_____

Information Packs

The compiling of information packs is one method by which important information you have gained about your patient can be collected and made available for others who work with him now or in the future. A collection of photographs, diagrams and videos will build up over the years to become a valuable record of considerable use and interest to those who meet your patient in the future. The majority of the multiply handicapped cannot speak for themselves and an information pack can serve as their voice to tell others about these patients and their needs.

Will you use information packs? _____

If *yes*, what information will be contained in them? _____

_____

_____

_____

Evaluation

It is extremely important to find out if your patient is benefiting from your work, or if changes are necessary. Without evaluation, at best you fail to prove that your efforts are worth while, and at worst you continue with treatment that is a waste of time.

You have already identified problem areas with your patient; these are already recorded in the assessment. If corrective or preventative treatment is recommended, it is necessary to record the results of that treatment. You may find that photographs and videos are useful for this. Physiotherapists use an instrument called a goniometer to measure joint range. This could provide you with objective information on the success or otherwise of attempts to prevent deformity. Doctors often use X-rays to provide a visual record of bone formation.

List below the treatments recommended and describe briefly how you will evaluate these treatments.

(to set the value

TREATMENT	EVALUATION

Looking Ahead

You have now completed *The Caring Person's Guide to Handling the Severely Multiply Handicapped*. In the Progress Chart that follows you will see that all the work carried out is directed towards building a firm foundation on which further work can be used. You will need to reassess your patient's physical needs and re-evaluate treatment regularly.

Now that you have established a firm foundation of good physical care, you will need continued and increased guidance and support from other professionals. In addition, you will have to plan further care reviews to cover your patient's social, emotional, occupational and educational needs and to find out how his complex needs may be met.

Key Worker's Progress Chart

In order for you to see at a glance how far you have progressed with this guide, please tick the relevant section of the chart below.

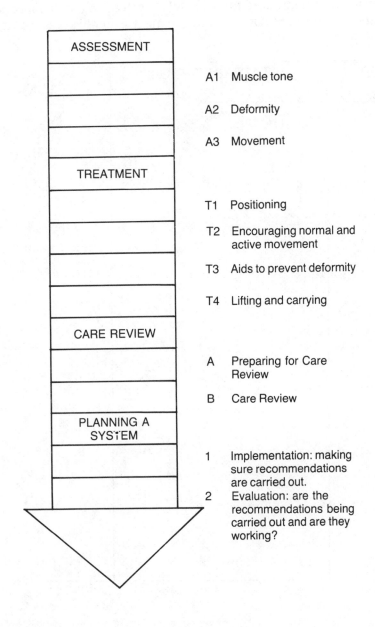

ASSESSMENT

A1   Muscle tone

A2   Deformity

A3   Movement

TREATMENT

T1   Positioning

T2   Encouraging normal and active movement

T3   Aids to prevent deformity

T4   Lifting and carrying

CARE REVIEW

A   Preparing for Care Review

B   Care Review

PLANNING A SYSTEM

1   Implementation: making sure recommendations are carried out.

2   Evaluation: are the recommendations being carried out and are they working?

A FIRM FOUNDATION ON WHICH TO CARRY OUT FURTHER WORK

Shopping List

Look through the guide and list any equipment that is needed in the space provided below.

Remember to bring this list with you to the Care Review so that you can discuss which items need to be ordered and how to go about acquiring them.

It can sometimes be difficult to obtain the necessary equipment for your patient. However, it is important to persevere because equipment which is directly involved in the therapeutic management of your patient is never a waste of money.

EQUIPMENT NEEDED	OBTAINABLE FROM	ORDERED BY (AND DATE)

Useful Further Reading

Finnie, N. R., *Handling the Young Cerebral Palsied Child at Home*, 2nd edn, Heinemann, London (1974). This book has become the 'bible' for those dealing with cerebral palsied children. It is sympathetically written for parents to understand but the information it contains is so important that it is invaluable to all those who care for such children.

Fulford, G. E. and Brown, J. K., 'Position as a cause of deformity in children with cerebral palsy', *Developmental Medicine and Child Neurology*, **18**, 305–314 (1976). This article outlines the importance of positioning and the powerful influence of gravity in producing severe deformity in children who are unable to move around.

Levitt, S., *Treatment of Cerebral Palsy and Motor Delay*, Blackwell Scientific, Oxford (1977). This is a comprehensive textbook on cerebral palsy and motor delay, written by a physiotherapist for physiotherapists. It brings together all the various 'systems' of management and contains ideas for, and rationale of, treatment, to produce an authoritative reference book and practical guide.

Perkins, E. A., Taylor, P. D. and Capit, A. C. M., *Helping the Retarded*, BIMH, Kidderminster (1976). When a person is both physically and mentally handicapped, those working with him need not only to know how to deal with the physical problems but also to have an idea of how to teach new skills and cope with problem behaviour. Although other professional assistance should be available (e.g., teachers, psychologists, etc.) to help those caring for the multiply handicapped with these issues, this book gives an insight into the subject by presenting the basic rules.

Scrutton, D., 'Developmental Deformity and the Profoundly Retarded Child' in *Care of the Handicapped Child: A Festschrift for Ronald Mackieth*, John Apley (Ed.), Heinemann, London, 83–91 (1978). This short article deals specifically with the problem of the development of deformity in children who are profoundly retarded in their gross motor ability and explains the best methods to prevent deformity.

This information is important to nurses, parents and teachers who work with the multiply handicapped, since many children are still affected by these problems.

Simon, G. B., *The Next Step on the Ladder*, 3rd edn (revised), BIMH, Kidderminster (1981). This book is written particularly with the multiply handicapped child in mind. It provides assessment procedures with suggested training programmes in sections including: use of sight and hearing; movement; manual dexterity; social development and personal contact; self-help skills and communication.

York-Moore, R. and Stewart, P., *Management of the Physically Handicapped Child*, pamphlets nos. 1 and 2, BIMH, Kidderminster (1979, 1982). These well-illustrated booklets provide simple guidelines to handling, lifting, carrying and seating the physically handicapped child.